A Record of
People
I Know
in Need of an
Exorcism

A Pastoral
Companion

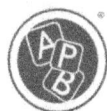

Angels' Portion Books

This Parochial Record belongs to:

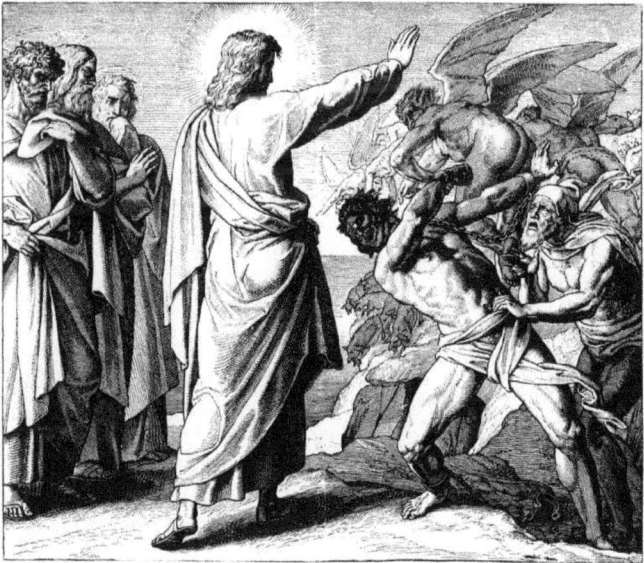

_____

"I've met the devil a few times. And each time our paths have crossed, while he rarely looks the same, there's no mistaking it's him. Funny thing is, he often resembles someone I know."

REV. CHRISTOPHER I. THOMA

Name:_____Date:_____

Evidence of Possession

Name:_____Date:_____

Evidence of Possession

2

Evidence of Possession

Name:_____Date:_____

Evidence of Possession

Name:_____Date:_____

Evidence of Possession

5

Name:_____Date:_____

Evidence of Possession

Evidence of Possession

Name:_____Date:_____

Evidence of Possession

Name:_____Date:_____

Evidence of Possession

Name:_____Date:_____

Evidence of Possession

Evidence of Possession

Name:_____Date:_____

Evidence of Possession

Evidence of Possession

Evidence of Possession

Name:_____Date:_____

Evidence of Possession

Name:_____Date:_____

Evidence of Possession

Name:_____Date:_____

Evidence of Possession

Name:_____Date:_____

Evidence of Possession

Evidence of Possession

Name:_____Date:_____

Evidence of Possession

Name:_____Date:_____

Evidence of Possession

21

Name:_____Date:_____

Evidence of Possession

Evidence of Possession

Evidence of Possession

Evidence of Possession

Evidence of Possession

Name:_____Date:_____

Evidence of Possession

Name:_____Date:_____

Evidence of Possession

Name:_____Date:_____

Evidence of Possession

29

Evidence of Possession

Evidence of Possession

Evidence of Possession

Evidence of Possession

Name:_____Date:_____

Evidence of Possession

Name:_____Date:_____

Evidence of Possession

Name:_____Date:_____

Evidence of Possession

Name:_____Date:_____

Evidence of Possession

Name:_____Date:_____

Evidence of Possession

38

Evidence of Possession

Name:_____Date:_____

Evidence of Possession

Evidence of Possession

Name:_____Date:_____

Evidence of Possession

Name:_____Date:_____

Evidence of Possession

Evidence of Possession

Evidence of Possession

Name:_____Date:_____

Evidence of Possession

46

Evidence of Possession

Name:_____Date:_____

Evidence of Possession

Name:_____Date:_____

Evidence of Possession

Name:_____Date:_____

Evidence of Possession

Evidence of Possession

Evidence of Possession

Evidence of Possession

Name:_____Date:_____

Evidence of Possession

Evidence of Possession

Evidence of Possession

Evidence of Possession

Evidence of Possession

Name:_____Date:_____

Evidence of Possession

Evidence of Possession

Name:_____Date:_____

Evidence of Possession

61

Evidence of Possession

Evidence of Possession

Name:_____Date:_____

Evidence of Possession

Name:_____Date:_____

Evidence of Possession

Name:_____Date:_____

Evidence of Possession

Name:_____Date:_____

Evidence of Possession

Evidence of Possession

Evidence of Possession

Evidence of Possession

Name:_____Date:_____

Evidence of Possession

Name:_____Date:_____

Evidence of Possession

Name:_____Date:_____

Evidence of Possession

Name:_____Date:_____

Evidence of Possession

Name:_____Date:_____

Evidence of Possession

Name:_____Date:_____

Evidence of Possession

Name:_____Date:_____

Evidence of Possession

77

Name:_____Date:_____

Evidence of Possession

Evidence of Possession

Name:_____Date:_____

Evidence of Possession

Evidence of Possession

Name:_____Date:_____

Evidence of Possession

Name:_____Date:_____

Evidence of Possession

Name:_____Date:_____

Evidence of Possession

Name:_____Date:_____

Evidence of Possession

85

Name:_____Date:_____

Evidence of Possession

Name:_____Date:_____

Evidence of Possession

Evidence of Possession

Evidence of Possession

Evidence of Possession

Name:_____Date:_____

Evidence of Possession

Name:_____Date:_____

Evidence of Possession

92

Evidence of Possession

Name:_____Date:_____

Evidence of Possession

Name:_____Date:_____

Evidence of Possession

Evidence of Possession

Evidence of Possession

Evidence of Possession

Name:_____Date:_____

Evidence of Possession

Name:_____Date:_____

Evidence of Possession

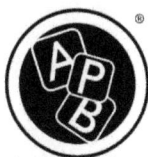

Angels' Portion Books

Please visit *AngelsPortion.com* for more
unique gifts for your pastor.